HELP

How to Help Those Who DON'T Want It...

by

Carol L Rickard, LCSW, TTS

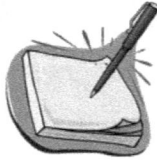

Sign up now!

To be sure to get updates, notice of
Q & A calls, and upcoming events
Text: HELPBOOK
To: **44222**

HELP!
How to Help Those
Who DON'T Want It....

by Carol L Rickard, LCSW, TTS

The ideas are the writers original and are an adaptation of Prochaska & DiClemente's research & model of change.

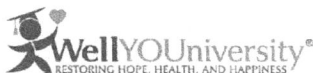

WellYOUniversity®
RESTORING HOPE, HEALTH, AND HAPPINESS

888 LIFE TOOLS (543-3866)

Carol@WellYOUniversity.com

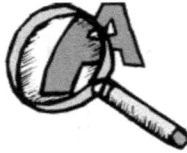

What will you get out of this book?

- A new way of looking at CHANGE.

- Increased understanding of HOW to be the best support to someone.

- Simple tools for being a healthy support.

- An introduction to "Selfness" & WHY you need to practice it.

Contents

Sign up now!

To get access to updates, more tools,

coaching calls, and upcoming events

Text: HELPBOOK

To: **44222**

Welcome

If you are reading this,

there are two things I know about you:

1) You have someone you
care about greatly.

2) You are feeling one (or all)

of the following:

frustrated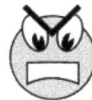

scared

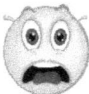 angry

These are very natural emotions to have

when dealing with situations involving people

who are close to us.

Maybe you're like me & have a loved one,

Who's been close to death & ***still***

doesn't see the NEED to change.

1

Or maybe you've been able to make critical health changes yourself & want another to make them too.

Or maybe you are watching someone who is **slowly headed** towards a train wreck and you can't get them to see what you do.

I am glad you picked up this book.

My promise to you is this:

You'll walk away from reading this material not only knowing HOW to **best help** another person make changes in *their* LIFE, but you will also be able to have some peace of mind by recognizing

what you **can** do and

what you ***can't*** do to help another person.

2

What this won't do:

It **WILL NOT** give you 'a magic wand'.

It **WILL NOT** get any person to 'change'.

It **WILL NOT** give you 'a quick fix'.

It **WILL NOT** even give you 'a fix'.

It will give you a
foundation!.

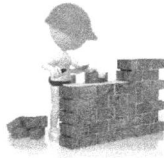

This foundation will give you the base
you need in order to be
the best support you can be.

About This Book

I doubt you have ever read a 📖 like this!

Unless, of course, you may have read

any of my **8** other books.

Along with **simple** & easy to understand

chapters, I tend to use a lot of pictures,

analogies, & word art

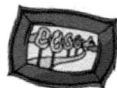

to make the information stick in the brain!

I call my approach:

SMARTheory™

It's what makes my books and services

different from all others!

KNOWLEDGE is the left brain at work.

This is where YOU *know* what to do!

Because I use "pictures" & "images", I end up
tapping in to the other side of the brain –

the right side!

This is also the side that synthesizes things,
like the operating system in a computer!

With both sides working on the 'same page',
the end result is getting people to

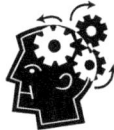

Move knowledge in to ACTION!

So, not only will you **learn**

how to help someone who DOESN'T want it,

you'll **USE** what you learn!

If you're not 100% satisfied when you finish reading,

let me know & I will refund your purchase price!

This book is divided in to **two parts:**

Part 1 will introduce you to my vision of change:

"The River Change"

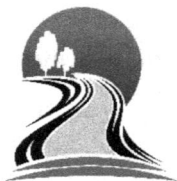

Here we'll focus on **WHAT** change is

& how to recognize where someone is

in their travels to The River Change.

You'll also learn the importance of

becoming a "River Guide"

By understanding WHAT –

You'll not only be the *most helpful* to someone,

you'll also be able to save yourself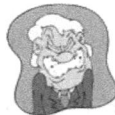

a lot of frustration in the process.

Part 2 we'll focus on the **HOW** to help

The goal of being a River Guide.is *NOT* to make change happen…

The goal is to help a person travel from one *stop* to another on *their journey to change!*

I will introduce you to the "tools" I've

used for the past 25 years to help people ......

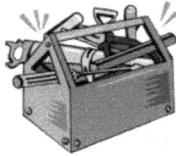

Here we'll focus on **HOW *to be*** &

HOW not to be *an effective* **River Guide**

These tools include:

COMMUNICATION

BOUNDARIES

MANAGING EMOTIONS & STRESS

SELFNESS

WHY I Wrote This Book!

There are **3 factors** that have influenced

my decision to write this :

#1 – I created a training this past summer to
increase staff's understanding of how
to **best help** their clients through change.

The workshop involved my desire to make

"change" **be a visual process.**

(you'll soon get to see this!)

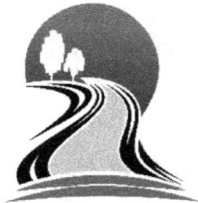

The workshop was a success!

Since then I have done the training for several

other groups with the similar results:

People are walking away with

a new approach to change they **can use!**

#2- I did a community program for a DBSA chapter. (Depression and Bipolar Support Alliance is a national support organization)

The program was for family and friends of those living with *a mental health condition.*

? When I asked people **?**

"What do YOU want to walk away with?"

It seemed their BIGGEST *need* was

"How to get somebody in to treatment

who doesn't think they need it."

There were some other things that came up too!

Like……

"How can I *say no without upsetting them?"*

"How should I *try to talk with them?"*

"How do I *get them to stop drinking & using drugs?"*

So I spent the evening answering their **?** 's.

It turned out **great** - for them and for me!

They left with answers and tools!

I left with knowing I'd given them answers

they so desperately needed!

The emails & 📞 I received afterwards

just reinforced how grateful

they were to *finally* have some answers.

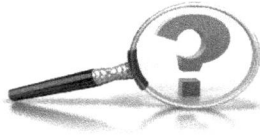

I came to realize there is a **great need**

for answers amongst family & friends of

those living with *behavioral health* issues.

The final factor is the crisis we are facing

#3- with opioids. There are *far too* many family

& friends being impacted by this epidemic.

There are *too many* individuals dying.

Just telling someone to

"Stop using drugs"

is *not* very effective.

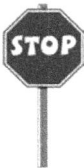

In fact,

It can sometimes have the **opposite** affect:

"Who the hell are *you*

to *tell me* what **I need to do?"**

I've heard patients say those

exact words

to staff in treatment programs where I worked.

If I can help 1 family member or friend,

learn to *support their loved one*

in a way to move them *towards recovery*,

this

will have been worth the time

&

effort spent writing it.

Why Listen to Me?

Over the past **25** years, I've had the

opportunity to help 1,000's of people

make healthy changes in their lives.

Many of them showed up for treatment,

BUT NOT because they *wanted* help

or

thought they had a problem....

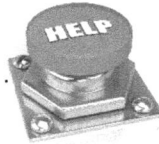

No,

they were there because *they had to be.*

For some, it was to avoid further legal trouble.

For others, it was to keep relationships
from ending.

And those, whose outpatient provider wouldn't see
them until they had 'completed a program'.

Using the tools & strategies I outline in this book,

I was able to help many recognize their need for

HELP & graduate from the program!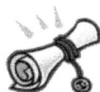

Early on in my career.

I learned some very critical skills.

I've also had the opportunity to learn

so much from the patients I've got to work with.

Along the way,

I developed some core principles &

strategies which have guided me to great success.

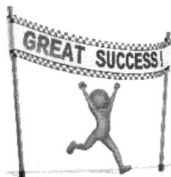

My approach has been shaped not just

by my professional experience,

but by my personal experience as well.

For there once was a time, in my own life,

when I wasn't in such a healthy place myself.

I was fortunate to be **"guided"**

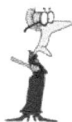

towards wellness and recovery.

In return, *I am excited to do the same for others!*

I have a Michelangelo

approach to health:

I believe:

We all have **wellness** inside us!

By giving people the right "tools"

& guidance on how to use those "tools" –

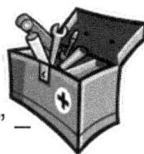

a person can **release** their wellness!

Just as Michelangelo

"released David from the block of stone"!

I have always dreamed of being able to reach

beyond the walls of a hospital

and help millions of more people.

I believe this is the mission

I was put on this earth to do!

I believe this is why I am

sitting here to write this book!

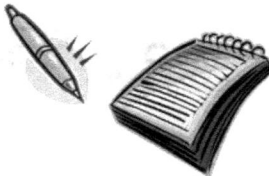

A Quick Check-In!

Just as I do in my live events, I want to have you

measure

to see where you are starting from!

Circle the number below each statement that best

describes where you are RIGHT NOW!

1) I think people can be resistant or in denial that they need to change.

0	1	2	3	4	5
not at all!					absolutely

2) I think all a person needs to do is make up their mind to change & they can be successful.

0	1	2	3	4	5
not at all!					absolutely

3) I can get so busy helping others that I forget to take care of myself.

0	1	2	3	4	5
not at all!					absolutely

Part I
The WHAT!

What About Change?

At my live workshops, I like to start out
with a little pop quiz!

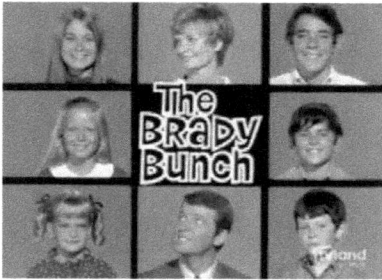

I call this:

THE SMART AUDIENCE TEST!

Raise your hand if you KNOW
that CHANGE *isn't as* **easy** as
the Brady Bunch makes it seem?

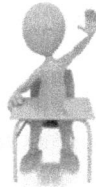

See, I knew you were SMART!

While I loved to watch The Brady Bunch,
the problem is that it, like most TV,
was not a very realistic representation.

Now, there is another example

I like to share with people:

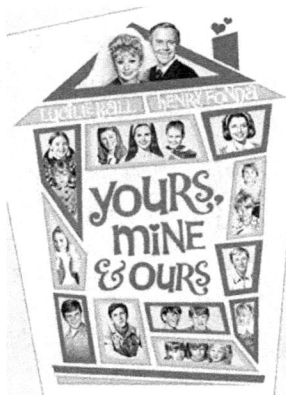

Yours, Mine, and Ours

This was a movie with Henry Fonda & Lucille Ball.

She had 8 children.

He had 10 children.

And as my favorite clip from the movie goes:

"*It was a typical wedding.........*

Enemies of the bride on the right,

Enemies of the groom on the left."

Definitely a much more realistic picture of CHANGE!

I grew up with a

Yours, Mine, and Ours

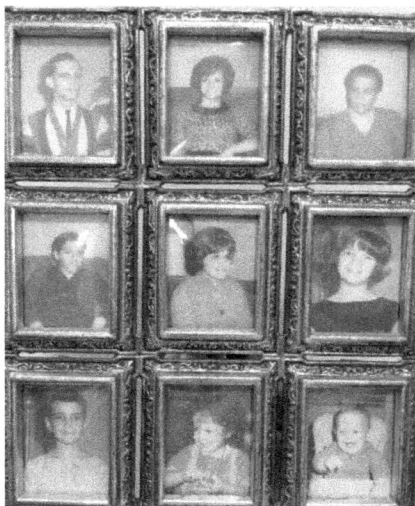

ME!

My father had 4

My mother had 3

Together they had 2
(Me & my brother Tony!)

And I can assure you, when the two families
merged – it was not Brady Bunch!

Change is not as easy as

'Making up your mind to do something
& just going about DOING IT."

It is a much more complicated process!

Since I started working 25 years ago –

I have always tried to

Make the Invisible Visible!

So I took this same approach to

Change!

The following chapters will take you

on a journey with George and

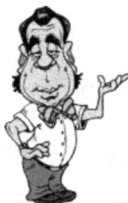

will help you to **SEE** change!

The River Change!

Imagine there's this river, "The River Change"

Life on the other side of the river
holds the promise of a *rich & happy life.*

However, the journey there
is not an easy one...

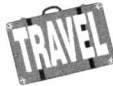

There are many people who set out
in their travels to The River Change –
only to never make it there.

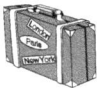

There are others who don't even

know the river exists!

And while a good number of people may never
experience life on the other side,

For the ones who do make it there –

the work of getting there was worth it!

Having a **River Guide** can increase a person's

chances of making it across "The River Change"

As we follow George, you will see

change has **less to do with his want & desire**

and

EVERYTHING to do

with *WHERE he is* in his journey!

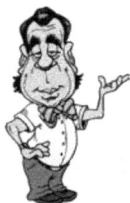

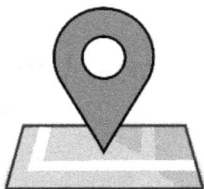

Where We Begin

George is a fellow who has some serious health issues going on.

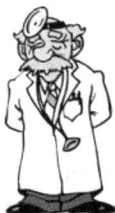

His doctor has **told him** he needs to "make some changes in his life" *if* he *wants to be around to walk his daughter Susan down the aisle at her wedding.*

Susan is 12 years old!

This isn't the 1st time his doctor has talked to him.

Last year,

George was HOSPITALIZED with chest pains.

He thought he was having a heart attack.....

Luckily for George –

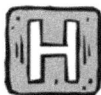

It turned out to be a panic attack.

George's wife, Sally, has been trying to get him to make some health changes since Susan was born!

She **told him**:

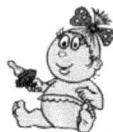

"I want you to **be around** for your daughter!

You see, George had lost his father when he was just **14** years old.

He then lost his mother at age **27**.

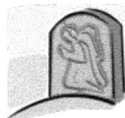

As it was, Susan was *never* going to get to know her grandparents.

Sally DIDN'T want Susan to have to experience the same **losses** as George did so early in his life.

Sally **THOUGHT** *this trip to the hospital* would wake him up.....

But it did **not.**

The problem is that George is in the

Land of Can't See!

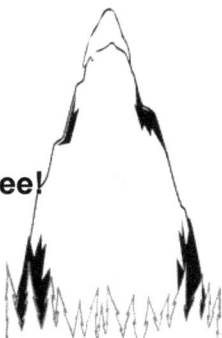

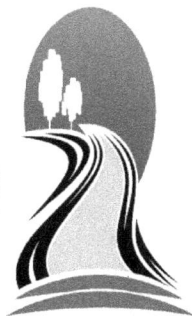

We can spend all the time we want talking to him about this river. The problem is:

George CAN'T SEE the river!

Take a look at the following illustration:

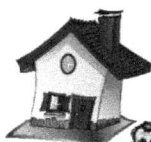

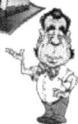

Land of Can't See!

WE can see the river very clearly!

From where George is – **he CAN'T.**

So if this makes sense, *we can't start talking to George about something he can't even see!*

He simply won't be interested.

I also call this "***The Place of Not's***"

When people are at this place, they are

NOT considering change

NOT aware there is a problem

NOT had any — consequences

In simple words –

They ARE **NOT** ready to make a change!

This is where a lot of people

will get it *WRONG!*

They keep talking to a person **AS IF** they can or they **SHOULD** see the river.

I've worked with a lot of patients, like George! They show up for help usually because they have been PUSHED to do so.

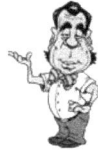

What I would hear:

> "If you ask me -
>
> I don't have a problem."

or

> "They told me I had to come,
>
> I didn't have a choice."

I think this quote says it nicely!

IT ISN'T THAT THEY

CAN'T SEE THE SOLUTION

THEY CAN'T

SEE THE PROBLEM!

GK CHESTERTON

Unfortunately, there are a lot of other words people would use to describe George being at this place:

Resistant

Denial

Unmotivated

Selfish

If we want George to have a chance,

then we must *get rid of these words.*

DO NOT USE THESE WORDS – EVER!

Resistant

Denial

Unmotivated

Selfish

Instead we should just recognize George

Is where he is!

One of my laws for success:

ACCEPT PEOPLE WHERE
THEY ARE...

NOT

WHERE *YOU WANT*
THEM TO BE.

CAROL L RICKARD

We'll talk more a little bit later about

HOW we approach someone who is in the

Land of Can't See!

It's not that we can't work with George,

or anyone else when they are at this stop....

We can! It just needs to match where he is!

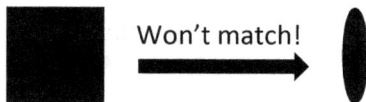

Won't match!

If Susan wants to stand a chance

at having George be successful

making these health changes –

she's going to have to follow my other law

START WHERE THEY ARE!

CAROL L RICKARD

We'll talk more about the **HOW** to help George, or
anyone else, coming up in Part 2.

For now,

It's really important to just *notice* where George is:

Land of Can't See!

? Do you **know anyone**
who's at this place? **?**

The Next Stop

After using some of the "tools" we're
going to cover in the next section,

Susan was able to help George move out of

The Land of Can't See!

Here we find George at the next stop in his travels-

The Plains of Potential!

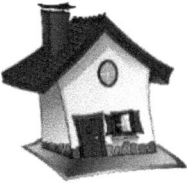

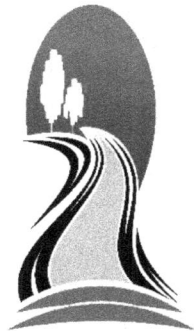

The Plains of Potential!

It is safe to say here -

We can see George has **started**

his journey to "The River Change"!

From where he is NOW –.

George CAN SEE the river!

I also call this "***The Place of Are's***"

When people are at this place, they

ARE seriously considering a change

ARE becoming aware of things

ARE looking at the pros & cons

In simple words –

They **ARE** getting ready to make a change!

This is also the place where people can

GET STUCK!

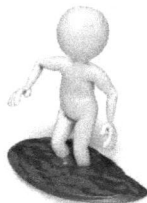

In my **25** years of working with people,

I've identified *a couple reasons* **why**

people can get caught & stay stuck here.....

They seem to ask themselves these **?'s**

- Can I really make it?
- Is it really going to be worth it?
- *What if* I don't know what to do next?
- *What if* I FAIL?

When I have worked with patients, who've
shown up for treatment where George is *NOW!*

What I would hear:

"I have a problem I think I need to work on."

Or

"I've been thinking I need to get some help for this."

Or

"I'm not sure, but I think I might have a problem."

Or

"I think I might need some help."

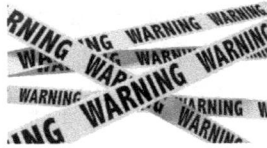

This stop on George's journey to the river

can become a very *frustrating one*

for those around him……..

He could STAY at this stop for a

VERY

long time!

In other words, their ambivalence takes over!

There's a story I read that illustrates this nicely:

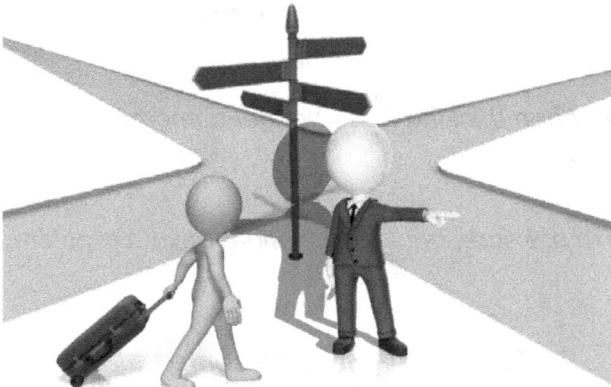

A business man was approached by a traveler
looking for directions to the **bus station.**

The business man gave him

very specific directions:

*"Go straight ahead 2 blocks & then
it's on the left side of this street."*

The traveler thanked him &
then headed off in the other direction!

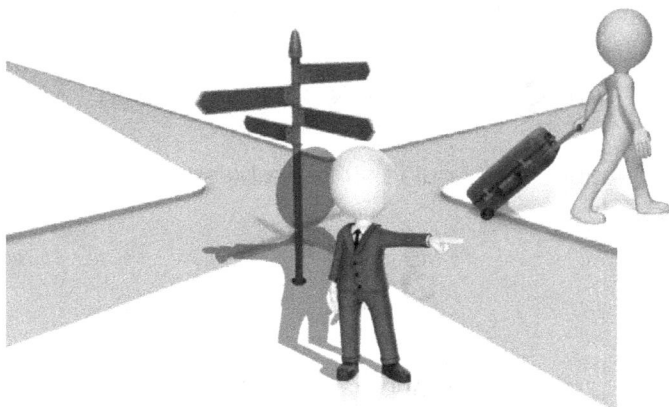

"Wait a minute!" the business man said.
*"It's the **other** direction."*

The traveler's response:

"Yes I know, I'm not quite ready yet."

The key to helping George, or anyone else,

who may be stuck on

The Plains of Potential!

Is guiding them as they find the answers

for those questions

&

Starting to help him build up the confidence

that he can DO IT!

The critical role for Sally to play here:

Become a *River Guide*!

A successful guide strikes a balance of the

3 E's

Encouragement

Education

Empowerment

(We'll cover these more in Part 2!)

The way I like to explain my role

as a **River Guide** to my patients follows:

"I'm not here to do the work for you!."

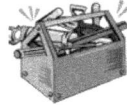

"I am here to give you the "tools"
so that YOU can be able to navigate life
SUCCESSFULLY on your own!"

I would also like to share a bit of wisdom

which was passed down to me when

I first started working **25** years ago......

DON'T EVER

WORK HARDER

THAN THEM!

Where To Next?

As George starts to make his way thru

the Plains of Potential –

he now finds himself at the next stop:

Packing Up!

George *IS AT* the river!

He's done a lot of work to get here.

but there is still more to be done

if he is going to get across that river!

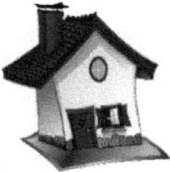

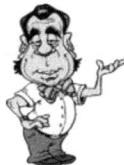

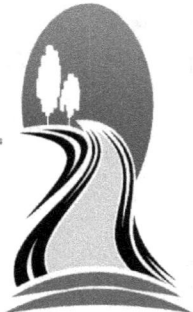

Packing Up!

Although Sally *wondered if*
George might ever get here,

she never gave up her hope or support!

I like to call this "*The Place of ...ING!*"

When people are at this place they are:

FOCUSING on a plan of action

IDENTIFYING their strengths

SETTING goals to move towards

MAKING commitments

In simple words –

They ARE **READY** to make a change!

This is where we can start to see

small behavior changes happen....

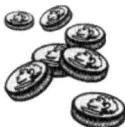

If you've ever saved

You know they can add up to BIG CHANGE!

The mistake most people will make here is

to look at these small changes &

fail to validate their existence.

There is **great power** in these small changes!!

An effective **River Guide** will be

on the lookout

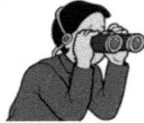

&

make sure these small changes

get acknowledged.

With George, Sally made sure to notice each time:

- George went to the gym
- Made better food choices
- Smoked less.

We have to be careful here!

We don't want to come off as treating

the person like a puppy or child either....

KEY POINT

One of the roles for the *River Guide* here is
to SEE & ACKNOWLEDGE!

NOT

TELL people WHAT to DO

For George, or anyone else, at this stop

in their travels to "The River Change"

there is effort being made!

If George is doing the work & nobody

around him is validating that effort……..

He could easily fall in to what I call the

Pit of F - it's'

'Why am I doing all this work if nobody cares?
F-it…..I'm going back to how it was.'

'Why am I doing this if it doesn't matter?'

One of the critical keys is

Validating the **EFFORT** & *not the outcome.*

Acknowledging the **BEHAVIOR** & *not the result.*

See the examples below:

Example #1

"I see you ***decided*** to stop by the gym."

NOT

"I see you *got to the gym*"

Example #2

"I noticed you ***waited*** to have a cigarette."

NOT

"I noticed you *didn't smoke*"

Bold = effort / behavior focus

Italics = the outcome / result

(we'll talk about more in Part 2 is HOW you do this!)

The other role of a *River Guide* here is

to ASSIST in the preparation.

This is a critical piece of success in the journey.

Without preparation –
George will be set up to **fail**

Once a decision is made to change, a person

must have the tools & understanding

to then go ahead with the change.

This could be any or all of the following:

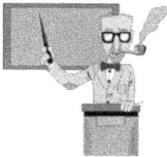

Instruction

Access to resources

Supplies

Examples of success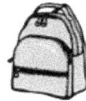

Support systems

Would you decide to *go white water kayaking*,

go buy a kayak & head straight to the river?

I don't think so……

You'll be ***more successful*** with a bit of training!

Are We There Yet?

It may feel like it has been a long time coming,

George has made it! (*Sort of....*)

He has left the banks of **"The River Change"**

and is now at.....

Making a Move!

Making a Move!

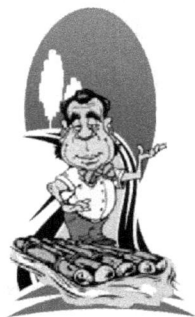

He is *TAKING ACTION!*

Take a look above at how far he

has come from where he started....

I like to call this "*The Place of DO!*"

When people are at this place they *DO:*

PURSUE the strategy they picked

MODIFY their behavior & environment

IDENTIFY with a new self-image

In simple words –

They ARE **DOING!**

This is where we can start to see

BIG action happen....

The mistake most people will make here is

to look at these **ACTIONS** &

see them as CHANGE!

ACTION ≠ CHANGE

Just like……

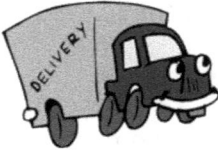 **⧣**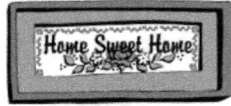

MOVING   MOVED!

There is a PROCESS

which must be completed!

Research shows it can take 3-6 months

of *DOING a behavior* (stopping OR starting)

in order for it to truly became CHANGE!

The example I like to use with my patients
is watching a house get built….

It isn't done in a few weeks!

Instead, each day they work on it,
the more it takes shape.

Until, one day it's finally a HOUSE!

Crossing

"The River Change"

Happens the same way!

Each day George works on the behavior,
the more it takes shape & substance.

Until one day it's finally a CHANGE!

The role of a *River Guide* here is

to SUPPORT & VALIDATE continued action.

This is a critical piece in order to have a
successful journey.

If George, or anyone else, stops

before they get to the other side....

It will become an experience with change

Rather than

A change experience!

They Made It!

George has finally **made it** to the other side of

"The River Change"

He is now at the last stop:

Holding Steady!

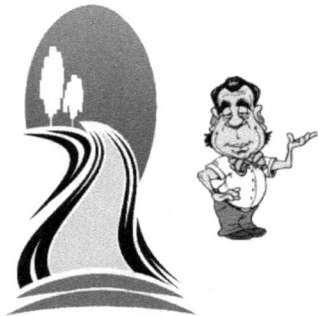

Holding Steady!

This may or may not be the final stop

for George, or anyone else……

You'll understand better in a moment.

It has been a lot of work to get here!

However, now that George is on the other side &

Holding Steady

The work must still continue..

I like to call this "*The Place of BEING!*"

When people are at this place they must BE:

SUSTAINING the gains

WORKING to prevent relapse

LEARNING to detect triggers & risks

In simple words –

They are *MAINTAINING* the change!

This is where we can start to see

Transformation take over....

Holding Steady continues

to be a lifelong undertaking.

Again, research has shown

the longer a person can hold change steady,

the more likely it is to remain a part of them &

the less likely they are to experience a relapse.

Even though they have made it across the river,

they still need a *River Guide* in their corner!

The role of a *River Guide* is to just continue to do

what they have done all along the journey:

ENCOURAGE		LOOKOUT
EDUCATE		SUPPORT
EMPOWER		VALIDATE

RELAPSE is lurking in the shadows.....

So now I want to talk about **WHY** I said

Holding Steady

may not be the final stop for George.

Have you ever been in a tornado?

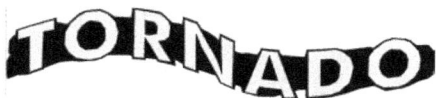

I have!

The scariest part about them is
how much damage they leave behind.

The 2nd scariest thing about them is
you can't do anything except

HIDE & HOPE.

You HIDE to avoid life-threatening injuries…..

You HOPE the damage will be minimal……

This brings us to:

Relapse Tornado

Relapse can strike George, or anyone else,

AT *ANY* TIME

Although it can happen at earlier stops

along the journey to "The River Change",

they are *most vulnerable* once they get to

Making a Move!

This is due to a **combination** of factors:

#1   Once **on** the open river, there is little place for George to hide, even when a storm starts to take form. (*Stress = Storm!*)

#2   Since skill level is still in the beginning stages, George might not be able to do much about it when the storm hits.

#3   Navigating through to the other side itself is a journey full of risks. Lack of experience can make avoiding them a little trickier!.

54

When I started working 25 years ago,

I was taught relapse wasn't just *possible* –

IT WAS PROBABLE....

Now,

initially I thought this was being a bit negative!
What kind of encouragement is that?

I soon came to understand it was no different
than with other life changes....

There is a learning curve

Think about it for a moment....

Did you learn to **stand up** the **1st time?**

Did you **walk** the **1st time** you tried?

How about riding a bike –
How long did that take you?

One secret I learned was this:

It's NOT *when* relapse happens but

WHAT YOU DO ABOUT IT

WHEN IT DOES!

The mistake most people will make here

is to look at **RELAPSE** &

see it as a NEGATIVE!

RELAPSE ≠ FAILURE

The critical role of a **River Guide** here is

to help George, or anyone else,

to see relapse as an ***opportunity.***

One of my sayings:

YOU *DON'T KNOW*

WHAT *YOU DON'T KNOW*

UNTIL YOU LEARN

YOU DON'T KNOW IT!

CAROL L RICKARD

If George views relapse as a FAILURE

It could take him ALL THE WAY BACK to

Land of Can't See!

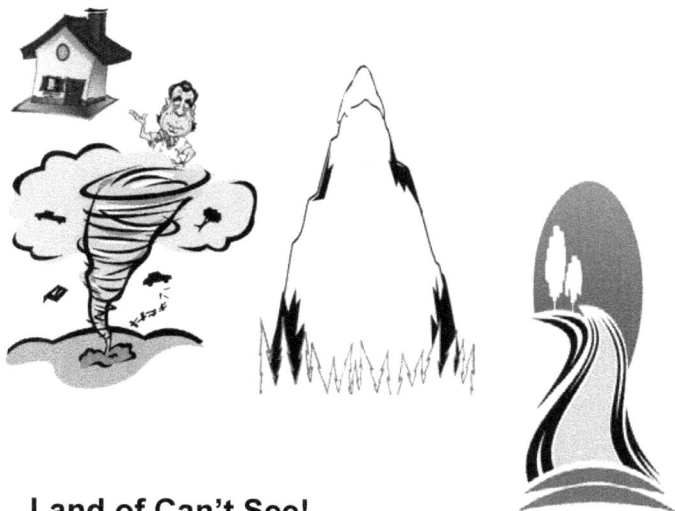

Land of Can't See!

In this case,

George, or anyone else,

will go back to the starting point,

And this is where we must meet him *again.*

If George views relapse as an **OPPORTUNITY**

It could only take him back to

The Plains of Potential!

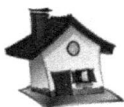

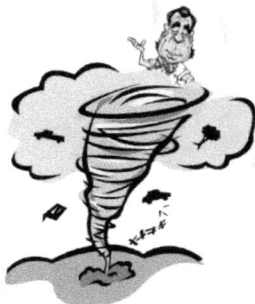

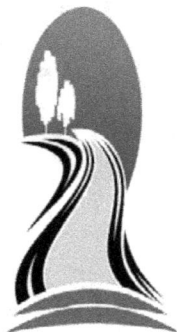

The Plains of Potential!

In this case,

George, or anyone else,

will not be starting back at the beginning.

Instead, they've landed where they can easily get

started on the journey back to the river!

Seeing CHANGE!

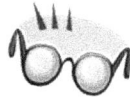

I wish I could say for certain that

knowing and being able to **see** Change

gives us enough power to

....Save people's lives

....See people succeed

....Eliminate life challenges

IT *DOES NOT.*

What it gives us is **at least** the chance

to be able to *help & hope*.

WE have **no more control** over another person

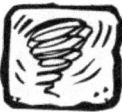

than we do the weather.

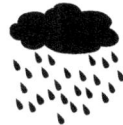

My goal is that by reading and putting this

information in to **practice**

you really are in a better position to

be able to HELP –

 the person *who wants help*

&

the person **WHO DOESN'T**

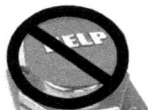

Here's the stops one more time:

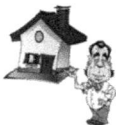

Land of Can't See!

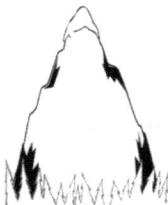

Plains of Potential!

Relapse Tornado!

Packing Up!

Making a Move!

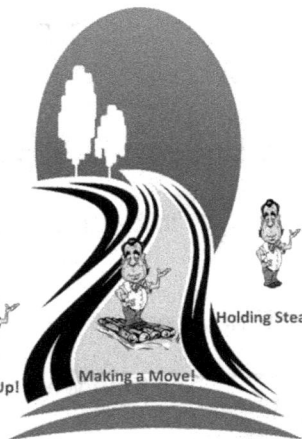

Holding Steady!

Part II
The HOW!

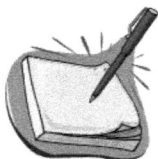

If you haven't done so already….

Sign up now!

To get access to updates, more tools,

coaching calls, and upcoming events

Text: HELPBOOK

To: **44222**

Getting Started

We focused on the WHAT so you can begin to
understand CHANGE in a whole new way!

We do not just wake up one moment
& decide we are going to

Make a Change!

There is a process to change – for all of us!

If we really want to help, especially the person who

DOESN'T want it....

1st   We must recognize WHERE
they are in their travels to

"The River Change"

2nd   We must ACCEPT where
they are in their travels.

3rd   We must GUIDE them,
not push them forward!

Our Foundation

I would like to take a moment &

revisit a couple of my laws from Part I.

Carol's RG Law #1

ACCEPT PEOPLE WHERE

THEY ARE...

NOT

WHERE *YOU WANT*

THEM TO BE.

CAROL L RICKARD

Or......

START WHERE THEY ARE!

CAROL L RICKARD

Carol's RG Law #2

ACCEPTING

DOES NOT MEAN

YOU AGREE!

CAROL L RICKARD

Carol's RG Law #3

DON'T TELL

PEOPLE WHAT

THEY

NEED TO DO!

CAROL L RICKARD

These are the critical foundations to

being an effective **River Guide**. **(RG).**

When we focus in these next chapters

on being a River Guide (**RG**)

the tools and strategies are for **US!**

Not any other person.......

If we go in to learning this information

JUST with the other person in mind

THEY WILL NOT WORK

There is a wonderful Stephen Covey quote

that sums up my point:

THE **GATE OF 'CHANGE'**

CAN ONLY BE OPENED

FROM *THE INSIDE!*

STEPHEN COVEY

So,

as you go through these next chapters,

do so with the intent on just becoming a better you!

The tools & strategies contained in Part II

can be utilized across *our lives*......

NOT JUST in trying to help

someone who doesn't want it.

After all,

the BEST **RG is the one who**

WALKS THE WALK

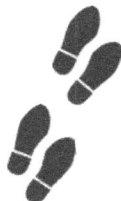

and not just

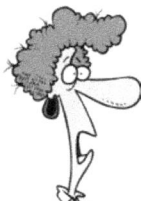

Talks the talk!

Communication

The Basics!

I'd like to start by reviewing some communication

basics which I've taken from my book-

"Transforming Illness to Wellness"

If I could teach only **1** skill to people,

this is it!

Let's face it – it's nearly impossible to get through

a day *without* communicating!

I believe the **QUALITY** of our life

is greatly influenced

by the **QUALITY** of our

communication skills.

It is **impossible** to be an effective **RG**

without communication skills!

There are **3** basic styles of communication:

Aggressive

Assertive

Passive

Aggressive: My needs and wants are all that
matters! It is my way or no way.

Passive: My needs and wants aren't important
at all. I'll just keep them to myself.

Assertive: My needs and wants are just as
important as your needs & wants are.

WAIT!

I forgot the 4th one!!

Passive-aggressive

I use to be the queen of this!

70

This is the **MOST** *DAMAGING*

to our relationships

Because it can leave us feeling they're

NOT BEING honest with us.

With this approach

Behaviors speak louder than words!

Examples:

1) Rather than *tell the waitress* the service was poor

I don't leave a tip!

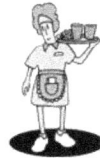

2) When you ask "What's wrong?" -

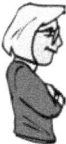

I say **"nothing"**

Yet, you can tell by my tone & body language

"something" is!

3) Instead of me *telling you I am angry*,

I slam doors & drawers, make a lot of noise,

or purposely do things to annoy you!

4) I communicate by **what I don't say**!

the silent treatment, showing up late,

or not calling when I'm supposed to!

It's like someone trying to SNEAK IN to your home

through the **BACK**

rather than walk in thru the front

Another way I like to have people
"see" communication:

Imagine we are both sitting at the table.

We are sitting face to face across from one another.

How would *you prefer* to be 'served'?

- I **shove** everything at you! (aggressive)

- I **set it** on the table in front of you so you can take what you want. (assertive)

- I **don't put anything** on the table, leaving you with nothing at all. (passive)

  or

- I set it in front of you then **take it**, pretending it was never there to start!

? Think about it… **?**

How do you '*serve*' other people?!

Communication is the single most important tool for **RG**'s!

Next, I am going to share with you my

6 Steps to Better Communication!

Talking Made Simple!

Regardless of WHAT approach you're currently

using, being a **RG** requires we be

Assertive

Anything other than this

will NOT WORK.....

It is critical that you start *practicing* the

6 simple steps I am about to introduce…

with co-workers

with friends

with neighbors & family

Practice them *away* from being a **RG**!

After all,

You wouldn't wait until you were on the **Titanic**

to *practice your new swimming skills!*

PRACTICE!

Here is my WordTool for Practice:

Purposely

Repeat

Activities

Critical

To

Improving

Core

Elements

Step #1

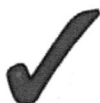 **Timing**

Ever had someone try to talk with you WHEN
your mind was *somewhere else?*

Don't make the same mistake.....

ASK first:

> *"Do you have a moment to talk?"*
>
> *or*
>
> *"Is this a good time to talk?"*

RESPECT THEIR ANSWER!!!

If they say **NO** – you can ask:

> *"When would be a better time for you?"*
>
> *or*
>
> *"Okay, I'll check with you later."*

The key here:

Don't push it! *No* means try again later.

Step #2

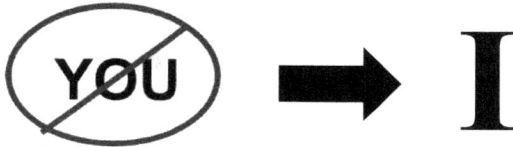

"YOU" is like an invisible **pointing** finger....

It's an attacking word!

Start all conversations with **"I"**

TRY:

I'm angry.

or

I feel like *I'm* not being listened to.

STAY AWAY from:

"You made me mad"

or

"You don't listen to me."

When people feel **less defensive**,

they **hear more** of what you say!

Step #3

????

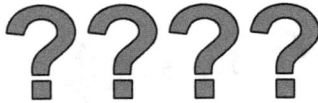

Ask a question, *rather than* **accuse**

TRY:

"What happened? I was getting worried."

or

"Is everything okay? I started to get concerned."

or

"Why didn't I hear from you?"

STAY AWAY from:

"You're late."

or

"You didn't show up on time."

or

"You didn't call me."

When people feel **accused** —

they *SHUT DOWN!*

Step #4

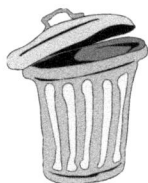

Always...never...everybody

They are fighting words!

When we use them, we **instantly** put people

on the defensive.

I call these **'trash can'** words.

Leave them in the trash can!!!

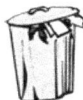

TRY:

> "**It seems** like we always go there."
>
> *or*
>
> **It seems** to never get done.

STAY AWAY from:

> "We always go there."
>
> *or*
>
> "It never gets done."

79

Step #5

WHAT DO YOU SEE?

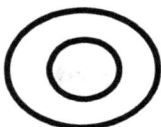

Tire	Lifesaver
Doughnut	Inner Tube
Cheerio	Bagel

Sure, we could *argue* about it.

The truth is we would BOTH be right!

2 people can look at the **SAME thing**

& *see it differently.*

We may not agree with that other person,

however, we must respect their position.

As I like to say: ***Agree to disagree!***

Step #6

THe Great EScape!

Finish off your sentence with

"......right now."

People are willing to *let you go now*

thinking there will be **a 'later'!**

TRY:

> *"I'm not able to talk about it **right now.**"*

> *"I'm not interested **right now**"*

STAY AWAY from:

> *" I don't want to talk about it."*

> *"I'm not interested."*

What *NOT* To Say

The **6 STEPS** you just learned will
apply across **ALL areas** of your life!

These are ***universal tools!***

Before moving on to more **RG** training,

I want to first share with you

What *NOT* to say.

They are the following:

You need to…

Why don't you…

Isn't it time you…

How could you…

What's wrong with you?

You should….

Didn't you know…

I don't want to…

What's your problem?

"I told you…

What TO SAY

Here are some things to *say instead:*

Help me understand …

How are you doing?

Is there a reason…

Have you thought about….

How's that working for you?

I was wondering….

I was thinking about you ….

I'm confused…

I am not able to…

"I don't know if you are aware of this…"

Again, I want you to imagine we are both sitting at

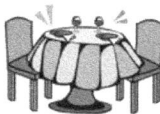

What to say = *putting stuff on the table!*

What NOT to say = shoving stuff
across the table at me!

83

Where to Now?

Now, we're going to take a look at each stop

& some specific tools & strategies **RG**'s can use!

Land of Can't See!

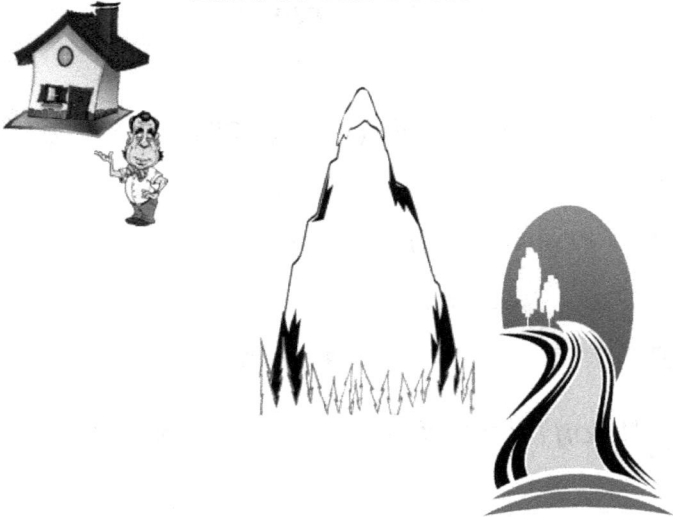

Remember, when a person is here -

they **can't see** the river.

So we *DON'T TALK* with them about the river!

Instead we want to help them

GET A PICTURE of where they are.

Here's a real life example:

A man came in to the ER having used *PCP*.

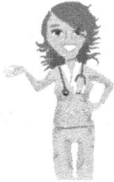

He was totally *out of control* –
saying his name was (unprintable)
He urinated & defecated on himself

He was **TOTALLY OUT OF CONTROL.**

Later, the ER nurse went to see him on the medical floor where he was taken once he was stabilized.

RN: *"Do you remember anything from the ER?"*

Pt: *"No, I don't remember a thing."*

RN: *"It was a mess!"*

Pt: *"What happened?"*

RN: *You kept saying your name was (unprintable) & didn't care that children were around. You urinated and crapped on yourself. It was a MESS."*

Pt: *"I guess I better **stay away** from that shit from now on."*

As you can see from the example.

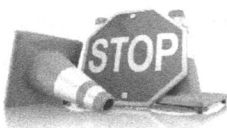

She didn't talk to him

about *stopping his drug use.*

She didn't *even mention PCP* or the word **drug use**.

Instead,

She **painted a picture** of where this guy was.

Read through the dialogue again to see

What else you notice she **DID or DIDN'T DO?**

(go ahead - this is important stuff!)

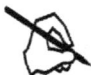

Take a moment & write it here:

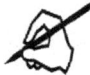

So let's review what she *DID* -

- She started out with **a question.**

- Used the ER as the **point of reference** — NOT *him or what he did.*

- Avoided using "YOU" until he asked *what happened.*

- *DID NOT* mention the drug.

- Stayed neutral & described *FACTS.*

- *DID NOT* tell him what he should do / not do.

- She *DID NOT* talk to him *right away.*

By just sticking with this type of communication,

we are better able to ENGAGE a person!

Use this formula:

A Neutral ? + "I" focus + FACTS observed

Let's see it applied to other situations -

#1 Family Function Drama

Don't DO this:

"You were drunk again." Or "You make a scene every time we get together as a family."

INSTEAD TRY:

(waiting until a day or even a week later)

RG: *"Do you remember anything from the dinner?*

JC: *"A little bit."*

RG: *"How do you think it went?"*

JC: *"I don't know why she always has to pick a fight with me."*

RG: *"I've noticed that each time there's a blow up alcohol is involved."*

Again,

we are just sticking to facts

&

putting it on the table!

Let's look at one more example -

#2 A Health Crisis / Situation

Don't DO this:

"You never listen to the doctor." Or
"If you cared about us – you'd take the medication"

INSTEAD TRY:

(waiting until a day or so)

RG: *"What did the doctor have to say?"*

JC: *"He says I need to take the medication &
need to quit smoking."*

RG: *"What do you think?"*

JC: *"I don't think it's a problem."*

RG: *"Besides going to the ER twice, what do you
think would make it a problem?"*

In this situation –

We are not saying it is a problem,

we're getting them to say when

THEY see it as a problem!

Moving to the next stop:

The Plains of Potential!

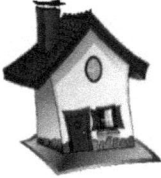

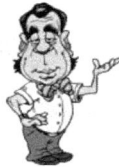

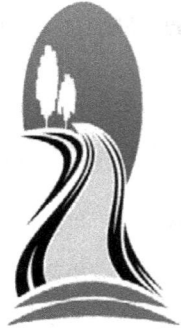

Here they are now *ABLE* to see!

RG's have to strike a balance of the

3 E's

Encouragement

Education

Empowerment

Encourage:

- **Look** for some strengths & **share** them
- **Acknowledge** the shift they've made
- **Call attention** to some of the +'s of making a change in their life.
- **Identify & validate** other times when they've been successful in their life.
- **Convey** your belief in their ability to change.

IMPORTANT: Don't *bring up past failures* or how many times they've tried this before.

Educate:

- **Identify & share** some +'s of change.
- **Assist** identifying potential resources.
- **Reinforce** change is a slow process.
- **Share** your experiences as they fit.
- **Collect & share** inspirational material.
- Take the time to **learn more** yourself.

IMPORTANT: Don't *come off as* the expert or Mr./ Mrs. know-it-all.

Empowerment:

- **Reinforce** the possibility of hope.
- **Validate** their effort.
- **Support** them doing *rather than* you doing.
- Continue to **build up** their strengths.
- **Magnify** the rewards of sustained change
- **Sustain** your belief in their ability to do it.

IMPORANT: Don't *give them* the fish, help them learn **how to** fish!

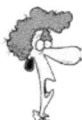

Things to say:

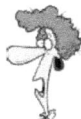

"I've noticed one of your strengths is..."

"You've made a great effort at..."

"Keep up the good work you've been doing."

"Let's see what we can find out."

"That's really good work."

"I can see you've..."

"How does it feel to have successfully..."

"I am so proud of the effort you've made."

"It's going to be hard at times – you can do it."

"I believe in you."

I can tell you've worked hard at..."

Another important task for **RG**'s

Pay attention to your own level of frustration!

I like to use *my feelings* as a mirror –

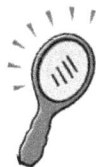

If I am feeling frustrated –
THEY are most likely feeling frustrated

If I am feeling annoyed -
THEY are most likely feeling annoyed.

Remember:

they can stay at this stop for a long time.

The more we can instill belief & *confidence,*

we increase chance of them moving forward!

The next stop:

Packing Up!

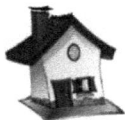

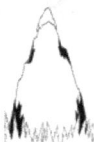

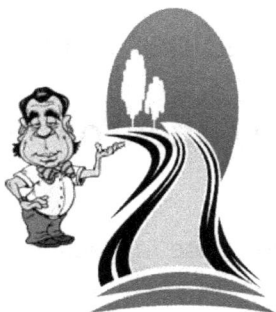

They are ready!!!

Of course we want to continue the $3 \; E's$

The **MOST** critical task for **RG**'s at this point:

SEE & ACKNOWLEDGE!

There's **effort being made** here & if we don't

1) notice the small stuff & 2) Say something

94

We run the risk of our traveler falling on to

Pit of F - it's'

This is where a whole lot of — self-talk comes up

& can start to **derail travel** to "The River Change"

Remember –   EFFORT

Here we're focusing on   &   **not outcome**
                                         BEHAVIOR

Things *TO SAY*:

*I **noticed** you .. (effort / behavior made)*

*I **see** you … effort / behavior made)*

***Great job** on (effort / behavior made)*

***Keep up** the good work on (effort / behavior made)*

*(person) **noticed** you (effort / behavior made)*

*I **hear** you (effort / behavior made)*

***Thank you** for (effort / behavior made)*

So here's some examples:

*"I noticed you **decided** to take*

the medication."

*"I see you **stopped** by the pharmacy"*

*"Great job on **reducing** your soda intake."*

*"Keep up the good work on **using** other*

stress tools instead of cigarettes."

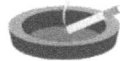

*"Joe noticed you were **getting** to the gym."*

*"I hear you **trying** to have better*

communication with your sister."

*"Thank you for remembering to **take***

the garbage up."

There are two other ways we can help –

1) *Continue strength building*

People can get so use to being **'criticized'**,
when they hear the *smallest of strengths* pointed
out **in them** they are eternally grateful!

[my secret: I focus on smallest success they've had –
example: person has very limited time of sobriety, say 1-2 days,
I like to turn this in to a strength]

The key is to be *genuine* or it **doesn't work**

2) *Assist identifying resources.*

Don't push – just set it on the table!

Have you tried…?

It might be helpful to…

It seems…

I was wondering if you…

Have you thought about…?

Change is a PROCESS!

How *RG*'s can help here is to

SUPPORT & VALIDATE!

I find the more we can validate

the work a person is **DOING** -

the **better** they *feel about themselves.*

This is important because it helps them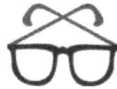

themselves in a whole *new way* &

the change

becomes part of a *new identity* for them!

This is critical for

long term success!

It's also important to remind a person:

Making **BIG** change in life

is like building a house –

it *doesn't happen* overnight!

Instead of focusing on how far they still have to go -

Help them see how far they've come!

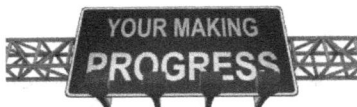

Things *TO SAY*:

Have you noticed how far you've come?

I see how hard you are working at this!

You are doing a great job!

Can you remember where you started?

You are slowly building a new habit!

I can see the positive changes you're making!

Can you remember how things used to be?

I am so proud of you!

Finally, we are at the last stop: (kind of!)

Holding Steady!

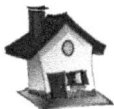

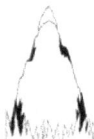

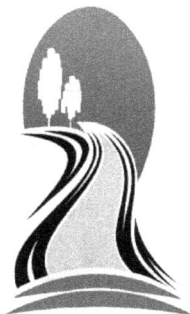

They made it to the *OTHER SIDE!*

Here they are *BEING.*

It's been a lot of work to get here –

AND the work must continue.....

They still need a YOU in their corner!

RG's are just as important now as ever....

The role of a **River Guide** is to just continue to do what they have done all along the journey:

ENCOURAGE	LOOKOUT
EDUCATE	SUPPORT
EMPOWER	VALIDATE

HOW we do this is using the same communications we've been using.....

Things *TO SAY*:

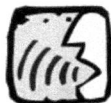

You did it!

I am so proud of all the work you have done to make this healthy change in your life!

How's it feel to ...?

Do you remember when...!

It's still going to be a little work maintaining it!

I know you have it in you to continue this!

Thank you for ...!

Of course.... what's lurking in the shadows is

Relapse Tornado

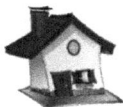

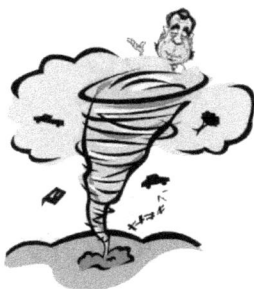

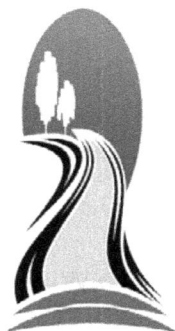

Relapse is a part of
the PROCESS of change!

The critical role of a **River Guide** here is

to help people see relapse as

an *opportunity.*

RELAPSE ≠ FAILURE

They work on the car –
fixing the problem.

We get back on the road & continue!

We don't go back & **start** all over again!

The same thing happens with relapse:

A person ***DOESN'T*** start all over again!

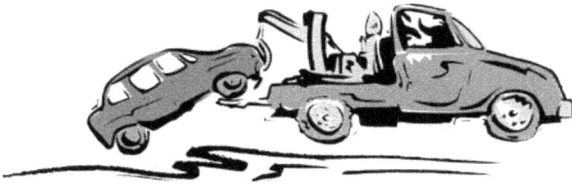

1. They **find** the problem

2. **Fix** it

3. **Get back** on the road

4. **Continue** where they left off!

The **key** point I try to

get people to **understand**:

Relapse happens!

It's WHAT we *DO with it*

that matters most!

Here is my WordTool for DO:

Direct

Opportunity

© 2017 & licensed by Well YOUniversity, LLC
Taken from "Words at Work"

I also like to remind people:

They didn't get walking down the first time either!

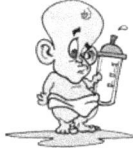

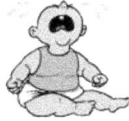

2) Learn from it

Sometimes a person might need **help**

identifying where they got off track &

even **seeing** they *ARE off track.*

I have found when people experience
a sense of failure...

They are at more risk for giving up

& going back to the

Land of Can't See!

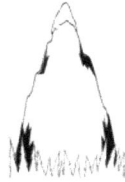

For those folks,

I like to use my WordTools:

Find
An
Important
Lesson
Using
Real
Experiences

Taken from "Words at Work"

And the shortened version:

F ace

A n

I mportant

L esson

The key is really helping a person see how
'falling down' can help us to learn & grow!

Boundaries

There are two ways we can do this:

1) Normalize it

People need to be **reminded** how

RELAPSE is a part of the process of

Change

I will often share my saying:

> YOU *DON'T KNOW*
>
> WHAT *YOU DON'T KNOW*
>
> *UNTIL YOU LEARN*
>
> **YOU DON'T KNOW IT!**
>
> CAROL L. RICKARD

An example I like to use with my patients
is taking a trip on the interstate....

There's a problem with the car.

So we need to ***pull off in to a garage***
at the next rest stop on the interstate.

Why Boundaries?

In my live events, I like to ask people to imagine for a moment, what it would **be** like if there were:

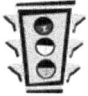

- No lines on the roads.
- No traffic lights
- No speed limits

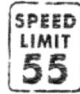

Then I ask them to shout out their answers!

I want you to write your answer below!

Now, think about how you would **feel**

If you were **not able to lock your:**

Doors

Windows

Cars

The next stop:

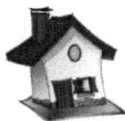

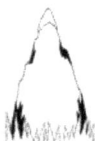

Making a Move!

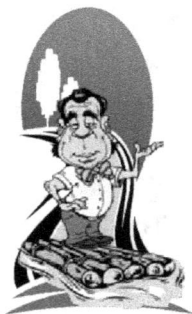

They are finally *DOING!*

While we may start to see

BIG action happen....

It is important to remember *this is not*

Change

The most common *be* answer I hear:

CHAOS

The most common *feel* answer:

UNSAFE

Right! We NEED those boundaries in our lives.

to help us *be* safe and *feel* safe.

They become a dividing line between

| What is
acceptable | What is
NOT
acceptable |

Just as we need boundaries

in our *physical world...*

We need boundaries

in our *personal world* too!

112

ME | **YOU**

NOT setting boundaries in our *personal world*

can lead to a whole BUNCH of problems:

- Feeling overwhelmed

- Getting taken advantage of

- Exhausted

- Manipulated

- Getting Sick

- Feeling used

- Trapped or Stuck

- Being an enabler

- Being a ***CARETAKER***

For *some people* this will be easy,

for others this may be *more challenging.*

I have an exercise I do that helps
people to quickly identify how *effective* their
boundaries are in their personal world.

To do this exercise, you'll need a volunteer!

STEP 1: *You are standing still* & your volunteer
stands about 4 feet away.

Pay attention to **HOW** that feels.

Does it feel "*comfortable*"?

STEP 2: You remain standing still & they take
a step closer to you & now 2 feet away.

Notice any difference? Still "*comfortable*"?

STEP 3: Keep repeating this, each time having
your *volunteer step closer to you*!
How does it *feel?*

Pay attention to *WHEN* it starts to feel

UNCOMFORTABLE?

IF you find yourself being able to

let somebody get *right up* in to your face,

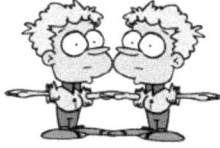

There's a very good chance you're at risk

for having **difficulty** setting

personal boundaries.

Only you will know this for sure!

The ***good*** news: This is a skill we can learn!

The ***bad*** news: You might need some

assistance to learn!

The most important thing to takeaway:

In order to be an

EFFECTIVE River Guide

We need to be **able to set** good boundaries.

Having **RG** boundaries means knowing

the difference between support

& *enable.*

The way I teach people the difference is to

ASK yourself these questions:

1. Is it something that makes ME feel better?
2. Whose responsibility is it?
3. Am I trying to do FOR them instead of them DOING themselves?

Support

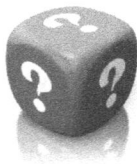

Won't impact my feelings

Is only *my responsibility*

Only DO for me

Enable

Makes me feel better

Is **NOT** *my responsibility*

I am DOING for them

Again, the greatest lesson I learned:

> # YOU CAN"T
>
> ## WORK HARDER
>
> ### THAN THEM!

A lot of times,

setting a boundary comes down to saying "no".

I'll be honest,

when I *first started working* at Hampton Hospital

I struggled saying "no".

Since I'd no other choice, I needed to keep my job,

I learned to **get better** at *saying it!*

Here's what I discovered:

My heart **WANTED** to say yes!

My head ***KNEW to say NO.***

I also learned that if I could say "no"

without actually saying N-O, it worked much better!

So here are some ways to do that:

I 'd love to, now just isn't a very good time,

I wish I could, I just can't right now.

Check back with me later.

Let me think about it.

I'll get back to you.

I'm not able to right now.

I'm afraid that's not going to work right now.

Can you ask someone else?

I wish I could, I don't have it to give.

Now is not a very good time, maybe later.

I can't fit it in right now.

Remember:

"**right now**" acts as the **great escape!**

Managing

Emotions & Stress

Managing Yourself!

One of the greatest challenges for **RG**'s is

being able to manage the emotions & stress

that go along with the territory!

So I want to share with you

a couple of my *favorite* "tools"

from a few of my other books!

1st

I'd like to start with a couple of my **Life Laws:**

Carol's Life Law #1

*You cannot **BLAME** others*
*for what **YOU** are feeling!*

We are 100% responsible
FOR OUR FEELINGS

Carol's Life Law #2

If we don't put words
to feelings –

***They come out
as behaviors!***

And lastly.......

Carol's Life Law #3

We have a right to
our feelings,

We *don't* have a right to
take them out on others

When it comes to STRESS –

My approach is like no other you've seen!

This good stuff comes from my book:

STRETCHED not Broken: A Caregiver's Toolbox for Reducing & Managing Stress

Do you have kids?

Has your washer ever been broken?

Do you hate to do laundry?

If you answered YES to any of the above, then you already may be a bit of a stress expert & not even know it!

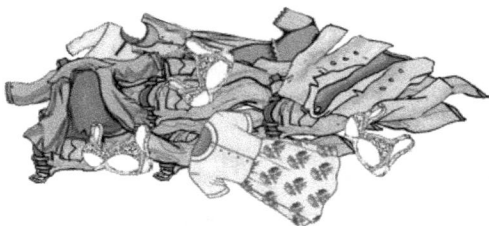

This is the pile of laundry after just 1 week!

Heading in to the next week, things are so busy
that you don't have any time to do laundry.
It has to **wait** until next weekend.

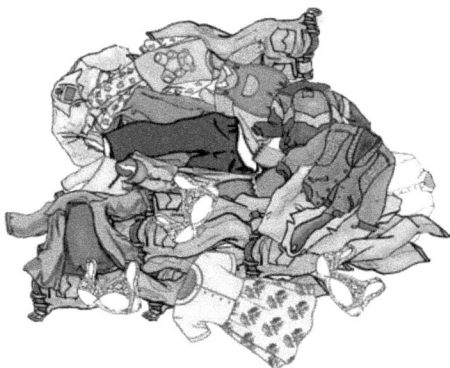

This is the pile of laundry you are looking at week 2!
It starts to GROW BIGGER!!

But wait.....

There just isn't enough time to get it all done.

You've got the kid's conference this week,
it's your mother's birthday, and
you still have to go shopping for a present.

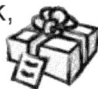

**Everyone has enough clothes to last them
one more week.....**

And there isn't anything happening next weekend.

So......laundry is put off for another week!

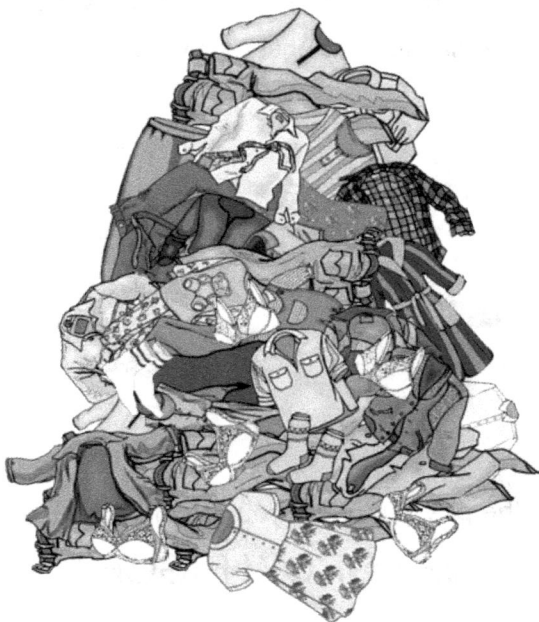

Imagine **how** you would **feel** if you had to look

at a pile of laundry as tall as you?!

What can we do to *keep laundry from piling up*?

Do a load as frequently as possible!

Sometimes we may need to do
2 loads or more a day!

STRESS is just like laundry!

It piles up!

Sure!

You can *pretend* it's
not there!

Maybe even try to hide it!

Whether you see it or not –

it still keeps *piling up*!

The solution?

Do **at least**
one load a day of

Stress Laundry!

LifeTOOL #17

{ This *means you must select and do at least
one of the activities listed in the following pages.
Don't rely on the same one or two.
Try things you've never done before!* }

126

STRESS AWAY

LAUNDRY SOAP

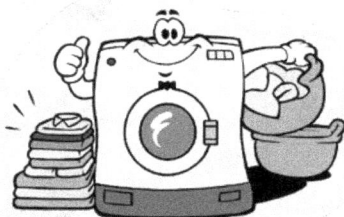

Guaranteed to lighten any day!

Directions:

* Use at least one time daily.

* Separate in to piles if
   too large for one load.

* May need to do multiple loads!

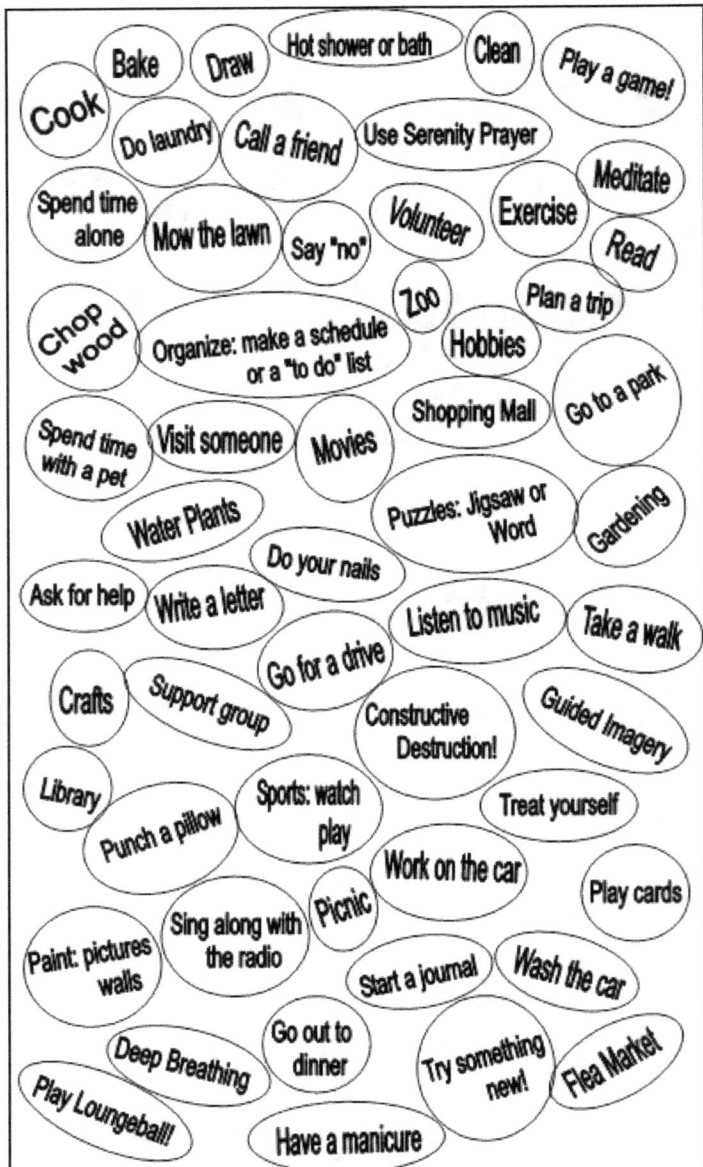

Bake
Draw
Hot shower or bath
Clean
Play a game!
Cook
Do laundry
Call a friend
Use Serenity Prayer
Spend time alone
Mow the lawn
Say "no"
Volunteer
Exercise
Meditate
Read
Chop wood
Organize: make a schedule or a "to do" list
Zoo
Hobbies
Plan a trip
Go to a park
Spend time with a pet
Visit someone
Movies
Shopping Mall
Water Plants
Do your nails
Puzzles: Jigsaw or Word
Gardening
Ask for help
Write a letter
Listen to music
Take a walk
Crafts
Support group
Go for a drive
Constructive Destruction!
Guided Imagery
Library
Punch a pillow
Sports: watch play
Treat yourself
Paint: pictures walls
Sing along with the radio
Picnic
Work on the car
Play cards
Start a journal
Wash the car
Deep Breathing
Go out to dinner
Try something new!
Flea Market
Play Loungeball!
Have a manicure

Another solution?

Avoid adding to the PILE!

LifeTOOL #18

Take steps to **AVOID** the things that cause you STRESS!

Only when I started doing my own laundry did I come to appreciate why my Mom would get so mad when I changed clothes a bunch!!

LifeTOOL #19

> # If it doesn't involve you
> # Don't get involved!
>
> Carol L Rickard

LifeTOOL #20

S + T = R

Situation   Thinking   Response

This equation is a **powerful tool** when it is used!

Let me share a personal example of this put to work:

One spring a few years ago, I was catching a flight back to Philadelphia from San Jose, California.

I was waiting at the gate for my flight when I **suddenly realized** the jacket I was going to need once I got to Philly was packed in the _suitcase that got checked_.

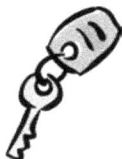

What made the situation WORSE was my car key was in my jacket pocket!

Now my immediate thought was "_I'm in trouble!_" (since we know how often suitcases don't arrive!)

My next thought: "I can't do anything about it now!"

I went back to enjoying the NBA Playoff game!

SITUATIONS will HAPPEN

What we **CHOOSE TO THINK** is a difference maker
migraine & no migraine!
stressed out or relaxed!

The Feelings Pendulum

What Do You Do
With Your Feelings?

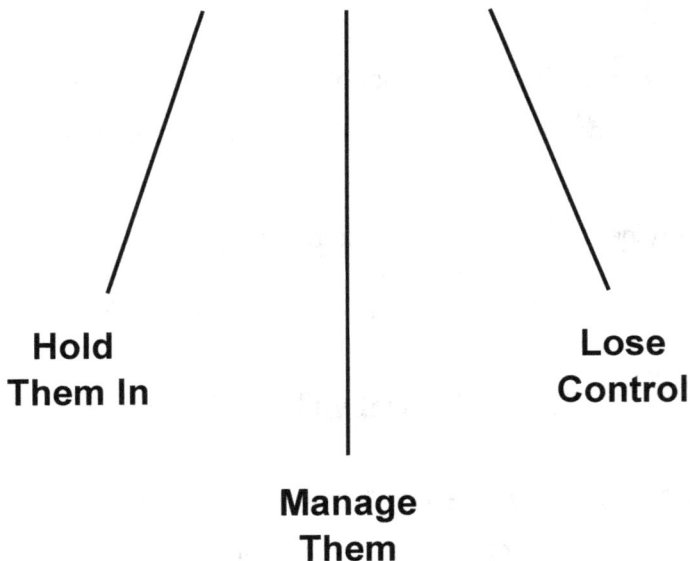

**Hold
Them In**

**Lose
Control**

**Manage
Them**

So which one did you pick?

If you are a "Manage Them", congratulations!
You obviously know what to do with your emotions!

If you are a "Hold Them In",
I am going to guess at times, you also can "Lose It"!

Finally, if you start at "Lose Control", & stay at
"Lose Control", **don't worry**! Help is on the way!

I like using a pendulum because it
perfectly illustrates just how difficult can be to

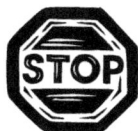 at "Manage It"

if you start up on either end.

Momentum makes it difficult to stop!

I have another way I like to teach people to
think about emotions and how to manage them!

First, let me ask:

"Have you ever said something
you wished had *never*
come out of your mouth?"

I think most people can relate to this experience!!

Here's **why it happens** –

When our emotions are so high that their level
is up to our nose – simply by opening our mouth
to speak they will come SPILLING OUT!

When things are at this **high of a level** –
we will have **NO CONTROL** over what comes out!

<u>Best not to say anything</u> when things are this high!
WAIT! There's an even worse level to be at....

BRAIN LEVEL!

When we are filled with emotion up above our 's we lose control over our brain!

It's like our brain gets **"flooded"** & we can end up

DOING STUPID THINGS,

not just saying them!

[Okay, maybe this hasn't happened to you. I'm sure you can think of other people this might describe!]

I have a simple process I teach my patients I call
Carol's Two Steps to Success!

Step 1) **STOP** the level from rising any higher.

Step 2) **RELEASE** so that the level will drop.

IMPORTANT:

It is only when the level is *lower* than the neck, *that we should attempt to talk!*

If our emotion is right at neck level it will *still* **CHOKE US!**

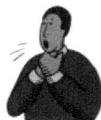

I have a few more tools I want to share with you!

How to
Live One Day At A Time!

My WordTool for TODAY:

T he

O nly

D ay

A fforded

Y ou!

First, read the following:

YESTERDAY, TODAY, and TOMORROW

There are two days in every week that we need not worry about, two days that must be kept free from fear and apprehension.

One is **YESTERDAY**, with it's mistakes & cares, it's faults & blunders, it's aches & pains. Yesterday has passed, forever beyond our control. All the money in the world cannot bring back yesterday. We cannot undo a single   act we performed. Nor can we erase a single word we've said – Yesterday is gone!

The other day we must not worry about is **TOMORROW**, with it's impossible adversaries, it's burden, it's hopeful promise and poor performance. Tomorrow is beyond our control!

Tomorrow's sun will rise either in splendor or behind a mask of clouds – but it will rise. And until it does, we have no stake in tomorrow, for it is yet unborn.

This leaves only one day – **TODAY**. Any person can fight the battles of just one day. It is only when we add the burdens of yesterday & tomorrow that we break down.

It is not the experience of today that drives people mad—it is the remorse of bitterness for something which happened yesterday, and the dread of what tomorrow may bring. _LET US LIVE ONE DAY AT A TIME!!!!_

(Author Unknown)

Then, take a blank piece of paper and write Yesterday, Tomorrow, & Today on it so it looks like this:

```
┌─────────────────────────────────────┐
│                                      │
│              Yesterday               │
│                                      │
│                                      │
│                                      │
│              Tomorrow                │
│                                      │
│                                      │
│                                      │
│               Today                  │
│                                      │
│                                      │
│                                      │
│                                      │
└─────────────────────────────────────┘
```

Under "Yesterday" -

I want you to write down all the things from **the past** (yesterday to 20 years ago) that still occupy your thoughts. This includes regrets, resentments, hurts, shoulda-woulda-coulda's, guilt's, & anything else!

Under "Tomorrow" -

I want you to write down all the things from **the future** that occupy your thoughts. Including worries, fears, "what-if's", uncertainties, hopes, & dreams!

Under TODAY -

I want you to look back over what you've written under yesterday & tomorrow. Ask yourself this **?** about *each* of the items you have listed:

"Is there anything I can DO about that TODAY?"

If there is, write down under **TODAY** the **SPECIFIC ACTION** you can take.

It must be something you can **DO!**

If there isn't,
don't write anything under TODAY

Once you have completed this,
there is one last step to take!

139

Fold the paper *just above* where **TODAY** is written.

Now, keep folding it back & forth several times on that same crease. You can even lick it if you want but don't get a paper cut!

Now carefully tear the paper along the crease.

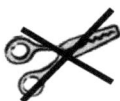

DO NOT USE SCISSORS!!!

It is IMPORTANT to do it by your own hand.

You should end up with 2 pieces of paper in your hands.

One piece has <u>Yesterday</u> & <u>Tomorrow</u> on it.

You *must* burn it, rip it up, shred it - destroy it!

The other piece has TODAY on it.

Hold onto this!

It is the only day we *CAN* DO anything about.

You may need to do repeat this every day until you're able to focus on TODAY!

140

The last "tool" is one which has served me well!

I am sure you are already familiar with it!

The Serenity Prayer

God grant me,

The **Serenity** to accept the things
I cannot change.

The **Courage** to change the things I can.

And the **Wisdom** to know the difference.

Here's how to use it:

Ask yourself this **?**

Can I *DO* anything about it right now?

If yes, *DO what you can!*

If no, you just have to **let it go!**

Leave

Everything

To

God's

Ownership!

Selfness

Taking Care Of You!

Before this book comes to an end......

I MUST introduce you to 2 last **RG** Rules:

#1) River Guides MUST practice daily self-care!

Or as I like to say

SELFNESS

This comes from my last book!

No River Guide has been known to

stay well **without** this critical practice

So, what is SELFNESS?

Many years ago,

I was running a therapy group

with patients at the hospital.

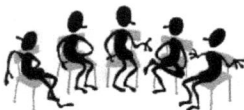

It was here that **SELFNESS** was born!

I had a patient I'll call Sue (not her real name!),
who was a single mom -

struggling & feeling overwhelmed

I asked her to identify **1** thing
she could do for herself tonight.

Her response:

"I couldn't do anything for me."

"I have to get the kids fed,
get them bathed & to bed,
& the laundry done."

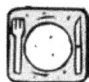

I gently nudged her to think of something

she could 'do for herself'

that would *fit around those things.*

Her response:

"I couldn't – I've got too much to do."

I'd spent several years working
in a women's trauma program.

One of the self-care foundations we used was:

The Oxygen Mask!

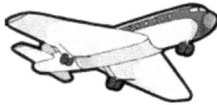

Since most people hadn't ever flown, I explained:

"When the oxygen masks drop from the ceiling &

you have a child or an adult who needs help –

Put the **MASK ON YOURSELF** first,

then help them."

Sue immediately stated:

"Oh I could never do that."
"I would put it on my children first."

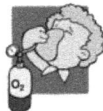

To which I responded-

"Then you won't be around for the kids,
because you'd pass out before you get yours on

& they can't help you."

Sue stuck to her answer: "I'd still do them first."

Huh? Her response didn't make sense to me so I
asked why she wouldn't put it on herself first.

She said:

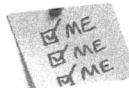

"That would be selfish."

I remember thinking

'Quick Carol, you've got to HELP her get this.'

Thank goodness my Higher Power helped &
I quickly came up with my own reply:

"NO, that'd be practicing SELFNESS!

which is very different from selfish."

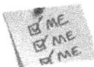

"*Selfish* is when we want other people
to do what we want.

SELFNESS is when

we *take care of ourselves* **1ST**

so we can be there to

take care of others who may be needing us!"

When I asked the group if this made sense?

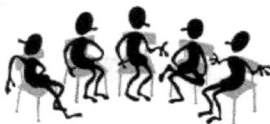

To my surprise, they all said yes, even Sue!

So I checked with her one last time....

"Sue, *who'd* you put the oxygen mask on *first*?"

She answered with a loud:

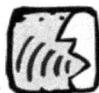

"MYSELF!"

And,

was born that day!

It doesn't get any **simpler than that!**

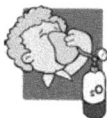

We MUST take care of ourselves

1ST

IF we want to be around

to take care of others!!!!

#2) River Guides MUST get support them self!

Being **RG**'s can be challenging at times.

Just as you are there to support the traveler, it is

equally important to have someone supporting you!

This could be:

- ✓ A support group
- ✓ A counselor
- ✓ A therapist
- ✓ A clergyman

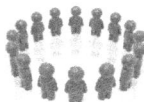

Think of it as having a look out party for YOU!

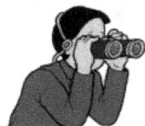

Sometimes *we can be* too close to see things

other people may be able to see.

&

Sometimes we need **new ideas** or

old ideas that *others have tried!*

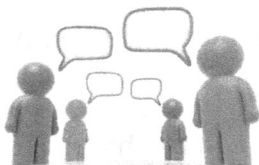

After all,

the Lone Ranger

did not fly solo!

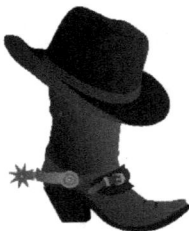

A Quick Check- Out!

So I said this would be again at the end!
Circle the number below each statement that best
describes where you are RIGHT NOW!

**1) I think people can be resistant or in denial
that they need to change.**

0	1	2	3	4	5
not at all!					absolutely

**2) I think all a person needs to do is make up
their mind to change & they can be successful.**

0	1	2	3	4	5
not at all!					absolutely

**3) I can get so busy helping others that I forget
to take care of myself.**

0	1	2	3	4	5
not at all!					absolutely

BONUS:

Send me an email with before & after scores!
I'll give you a 30-minute coaching call with me!!!

Carol@WellYOUniversity.com   Subject: HELP!
Limited number of slots available!

About the Author

Carol L Rickard, LCSW, TTS, of Hopewell, NJ is founder & CEO of WellYOUniversity, LLC, a global health education company dedicated *to empowering individuals with the tools and supports to achieve lifelong wellness & recovery.*

Also known as **America's Wellness Ambassador**, Carol is a dynamic & engaging speaker who brings to life practical / useful solutions. She is a weekly contributor for Esperanza Magazine; written 13 books on stress and wellness, had a guest appearance on Dr. Oz last year

She is also the creator & host of a 30-minute wellness show on Princeton TV - **The WELL YOU Show** which can be seen at:

www.vimeo.com/channels/wellyou

Get more of Carol at:

Twitter: **@wellYOUlife**

"Like us" @ www.FaceBook.com/WellYOUniversity

Have Carol Speak at Your Next Event!

Get more information about how you can have Carol speak at your organization, event, or conference.

Go to: www.CarolLRickard.com

Or call: 888 Life Tools (543-3866)

Carol's Other Books

Selfness

Stress Eating

Stretched Not Broken

The Caregiver's Toolbox

Transforming Illness to Wellness

Putting Your Weight Loss on Auto

The Benefits of Smoking

Moving Beyond Depression

LifeTools

Words At Work Vol. 1

Words at Work Vol. 2

Creating Compliance

Relapse Prevention

Please visit us at:

www.WellYOUniversity.com

Sign up for weekly motivational e-quote!

Check out our upcoming FREE webinars!

Learn more about our training programs.

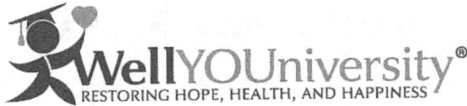

WellYOUniversity®
RESTORING HOPE, HEALTH, AND HAPPINESS

Email us your success story at:

Success@WellYOUniversity.com

We'd like to ask for your feedback

Please check out the last page
if this book has been HELPFUL for you!

We'd love to hear from you!

Feedback Card

Please take a moment & provide us some
feedback about the book you just read &
how you feel *it benefited YOU!*

_____

_____

_____

_____

Name: _____

Best Phone #: _____

Can we use your comments in our publicity materials?

Yes / No

If OK with you, what's the best time to call you:_____

Thank You!

Scan or take a picture & email:

Carol@WellYOUniversity.com

Snail mail:　　　　Carol Rickard

5 Zion Rd., Hopewell, NJ 08535

155